30-DAY
SOCIAL MEDIA
DETOX

DAY 1

- [ ] No Facebook until 12pm.

HOW DO YOU FEEL?

☐ Delete all unused apps.

HOW DO YOU FEEL?

DAY 3

- [ ] No social media updates today!

HOW DO YOU FEEL?

No phone during meal times.

HOW DO YOU FEEL?

DAY 5

☐ No social media scrolling till 11am.

HOW DO YOU FEEL?

DAY 6

- [ ] Call a friend today— don't just stalk.

HOW DO YOU FEEL?

DAY 7

- [ ] **Twitter free day!**

HOW DO YOU FEEL?

DAY 8

- [ ] Meditate 15-20min Phone free.

HOW DO YOU FEEL?

- [ ] Put your phone in a seperate room at bedtime.

HOW DO YOU FEEL?

DAY 10

- [ ] Spend 2h phone free with someone.

HOW DO YOU FEEL?

DAY 11

☐ No
Facebook
all day!

HOW DO YOU FEEL?

DAY 12

- [ ] Limit of 20min social media today.

HOW DO YOU FEEL?

HOW DO YOU FEEL?

- [ ] No status updates today!

HOW DO YOU FEEL?

DAY 14

- [ ] Walk for 1h outside.

HOW DO YOU FEEL?

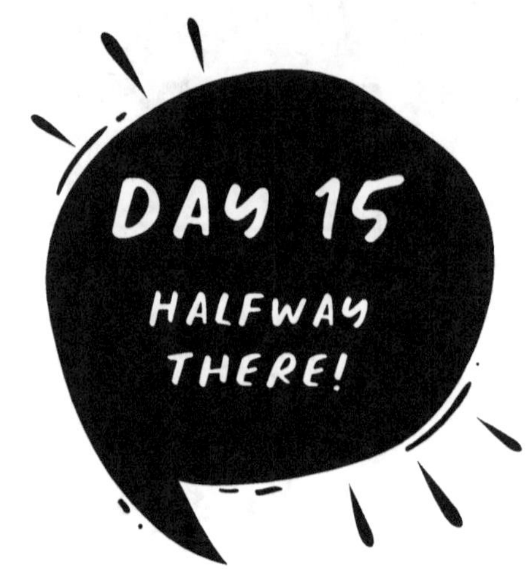

☐ **No social media all day!**

HOW DO YOU FEEL?

DAY 16

☐ **No phone at meals all day!**

HOW DO YOU FEEL?

DAY 17

☐ Laptop & phone off by 6pm.

HOW DO YOU FEEL?

DAY 18

- [ ] 30min social media limit.

HOW DO YOU FEEL?

DAY 19

- Exercise phone free today.

HOW DO YOU FEEL?

DAY 20

☐ # No Insta all day!

HOW DO YOU FEEL?

DAY 21

- [ ] 20min social media limit.

HOW DO YOU FEEL?

DAY 22

☐ Read a book for 45min.

HOW DO YOU FEEL?

DAY 23

- [ ] No social media scrolling till 3pm.

HOW DO YOU FEEL?

DAY 24

- [ ] No social media after 5pm.

HOW DO YOU FEEL?

DAY 25

- [ ] 15min social media limit.

HOW DO YOU FEEL?

DAY 26

- [ ] Zero social media today.

HOW DO YOU FEEL?

DAY 27

Suprise a loved one. No phone today.

HOW DO YOU FEEL?

☐ No phone after work/ school.

HOW DO YOU FEEL?

DAY 29

- [ ] Set up future goals. No phone for 1h.

HOW DO YOU FEEL?

DAY 30

☐ Your choice— challenge yourself!

HOW DO YOU FEEL?

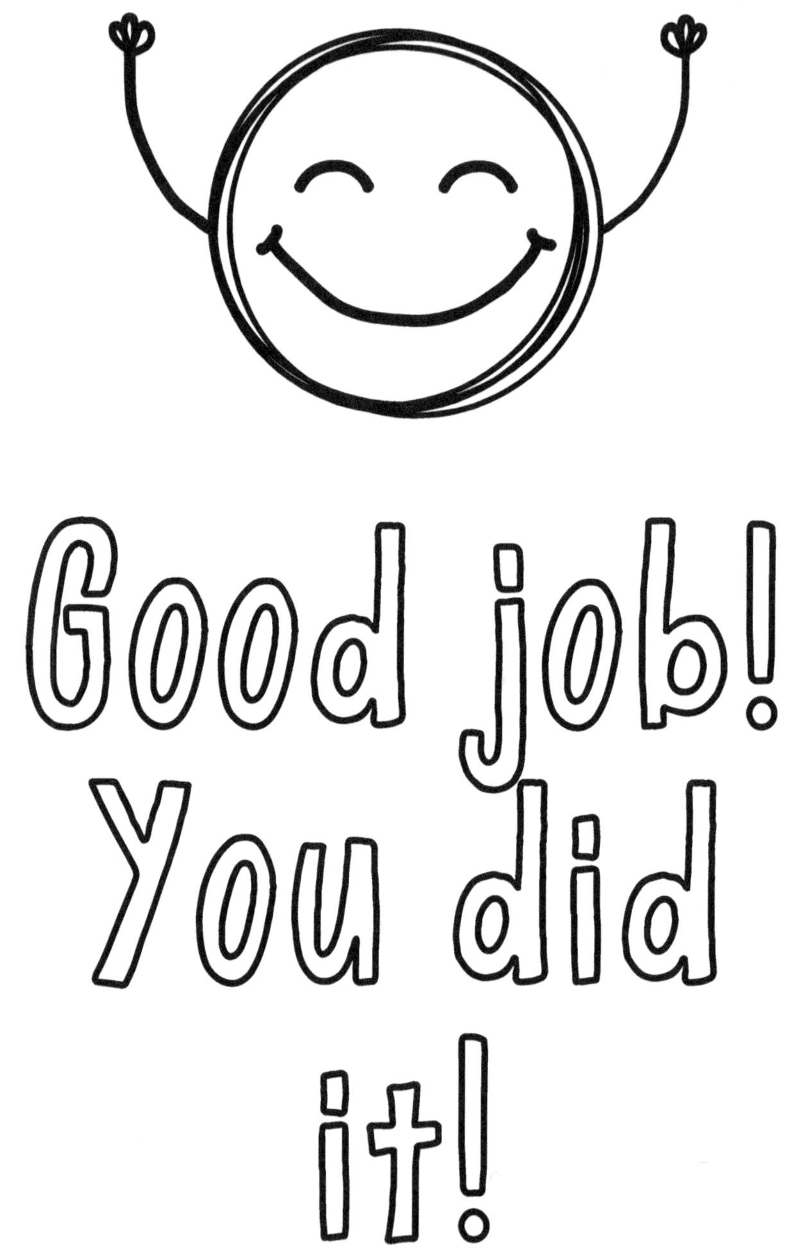
Good job!
You did
it!

HOW DO YOU FEEL?

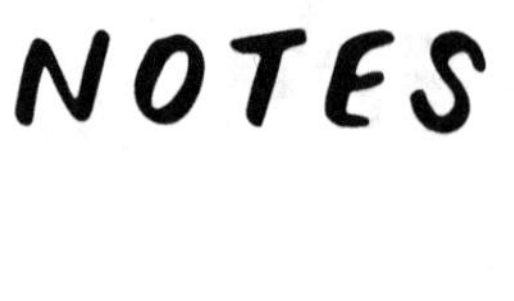

NOTES

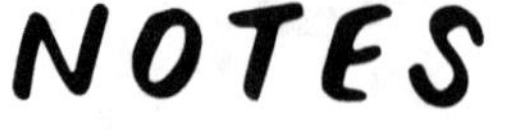

NOTES

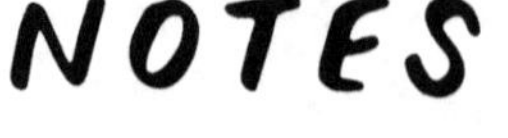

NOTES

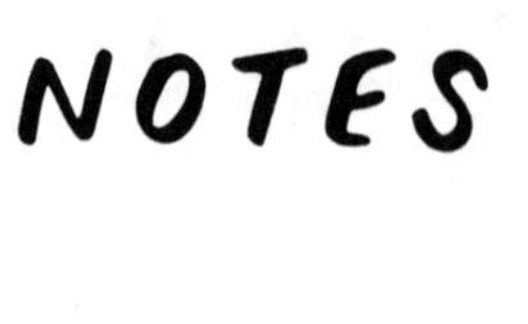

NOTES

NOTES

NOTES

NOTES

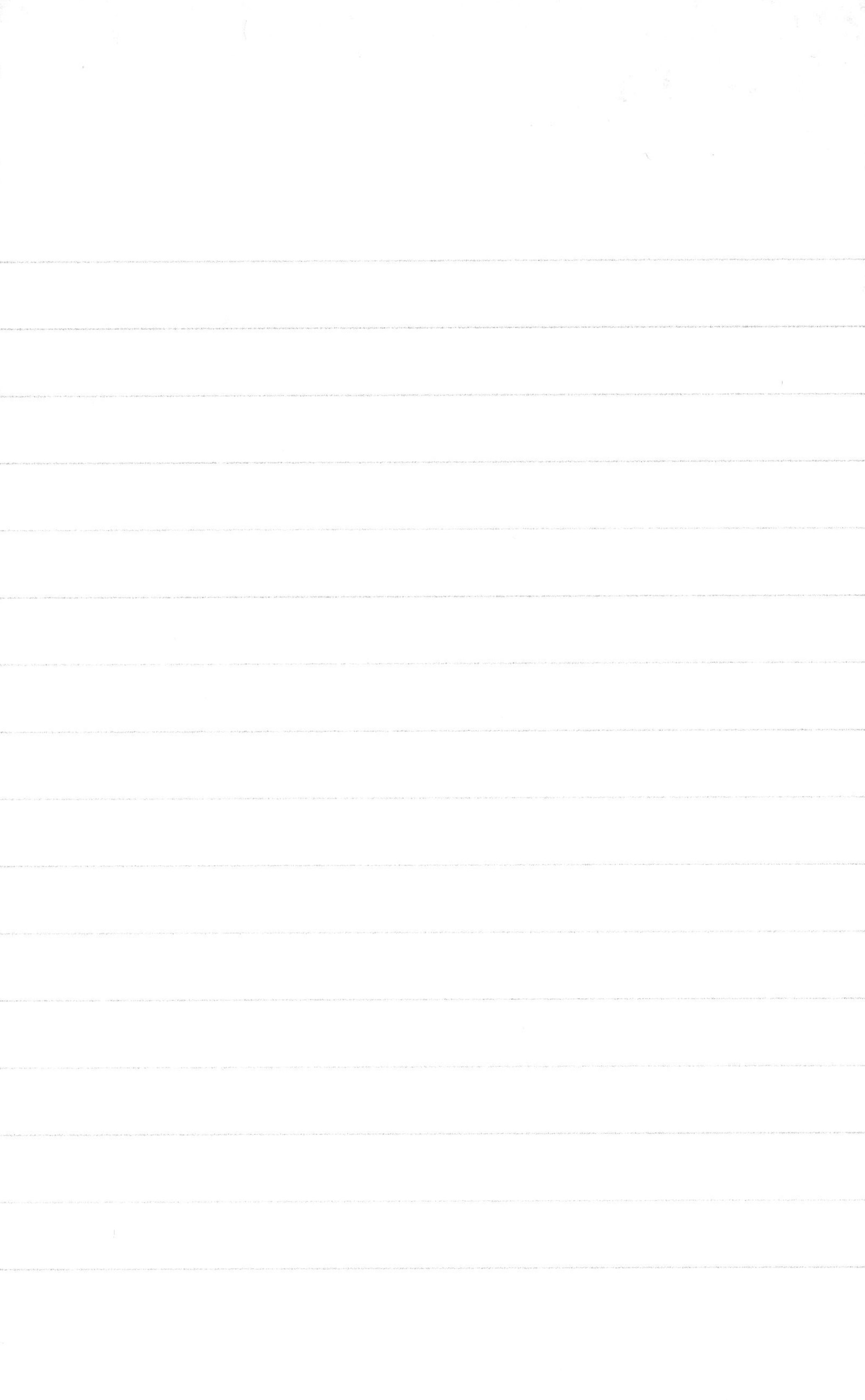

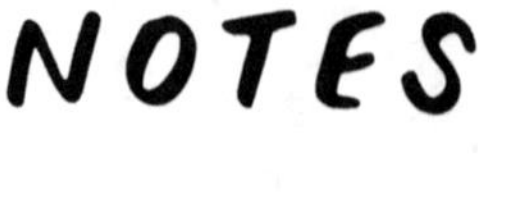

NOTES

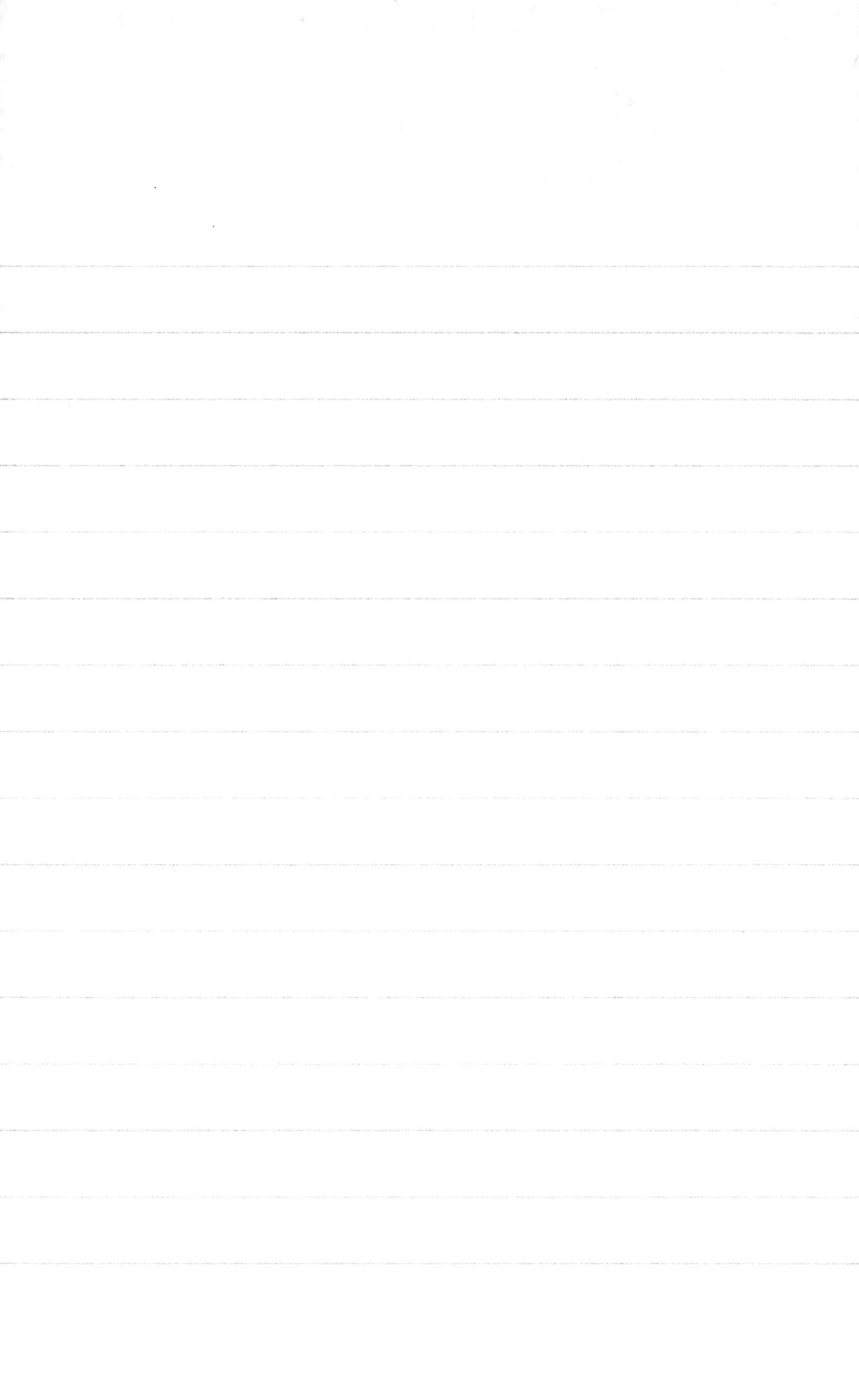

NOTES

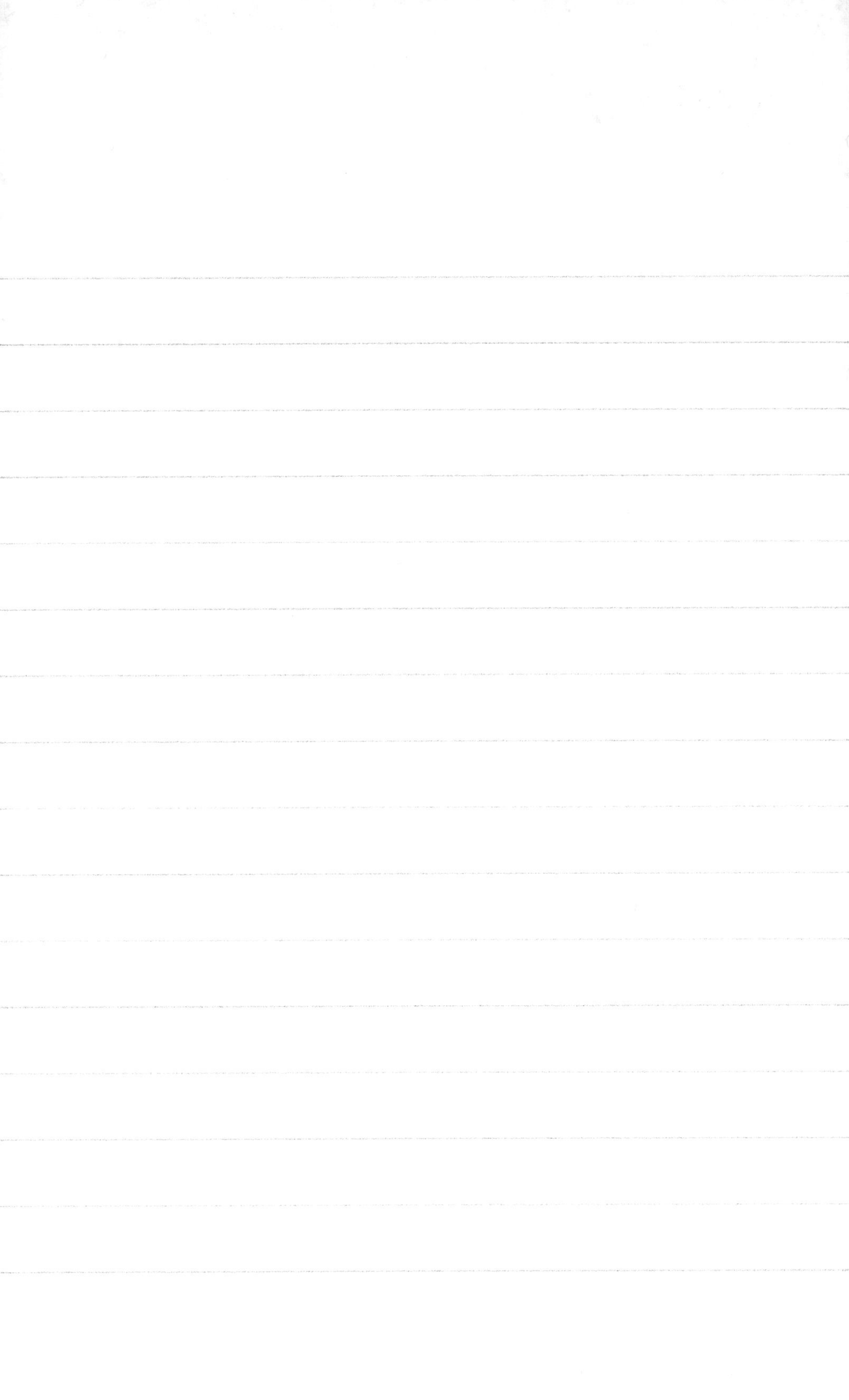

NOTES

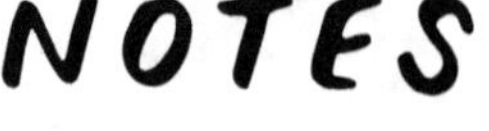

NOTES

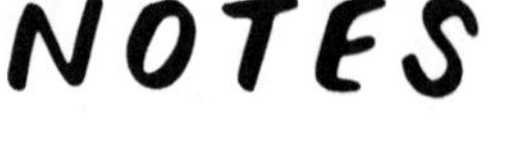

NOTES

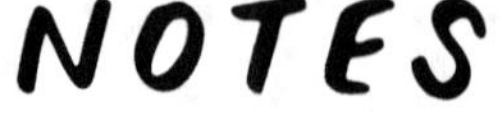

NOTES

NOTES

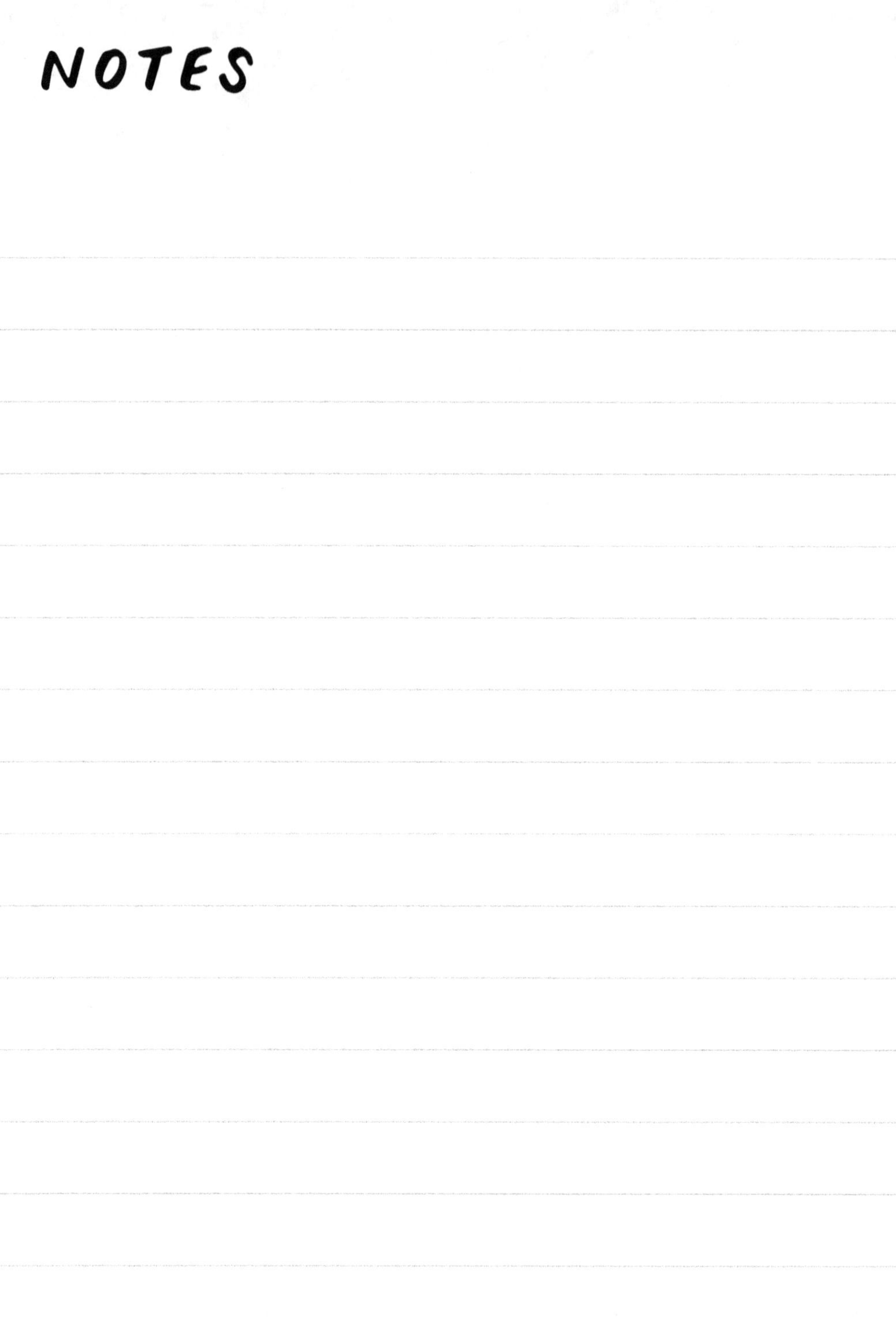

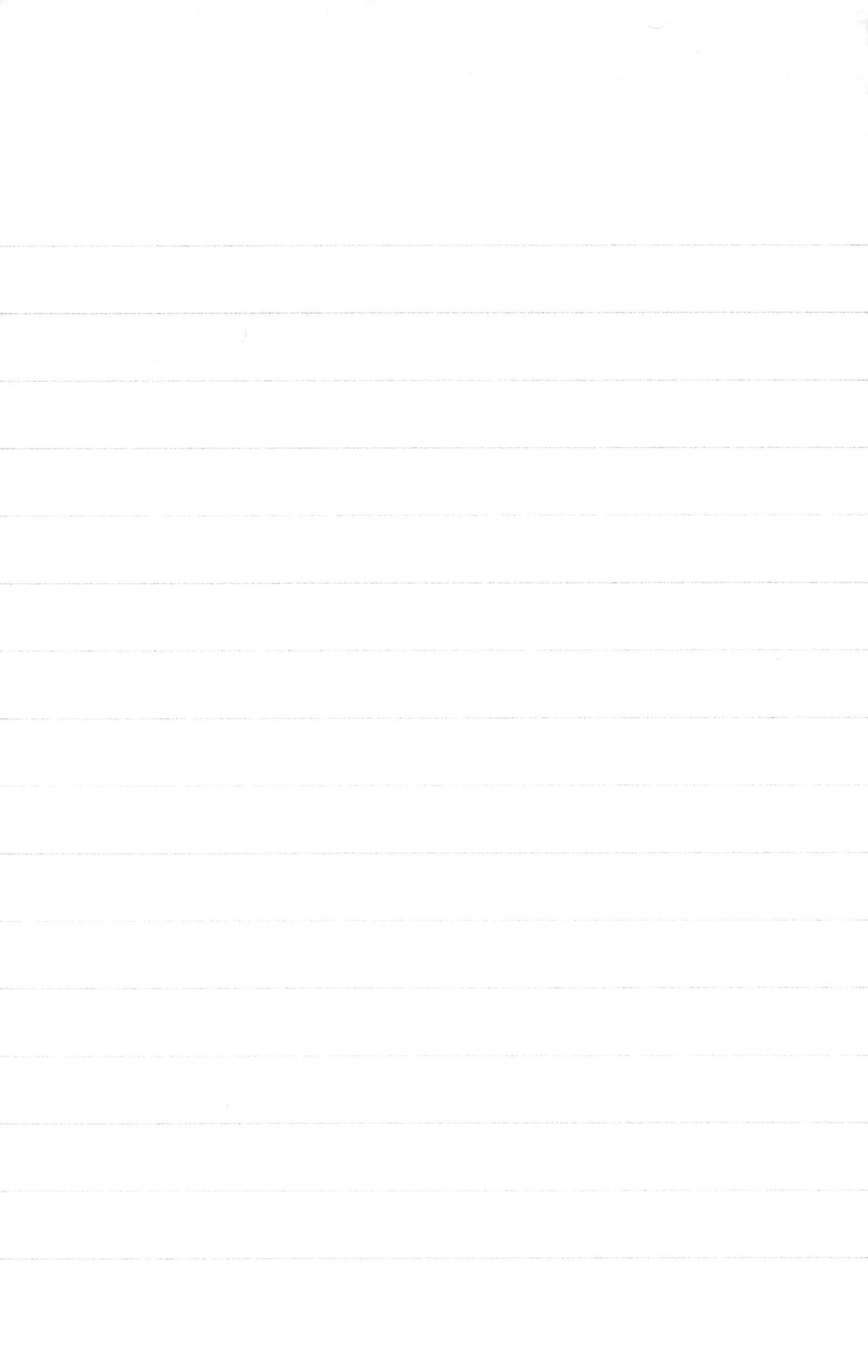

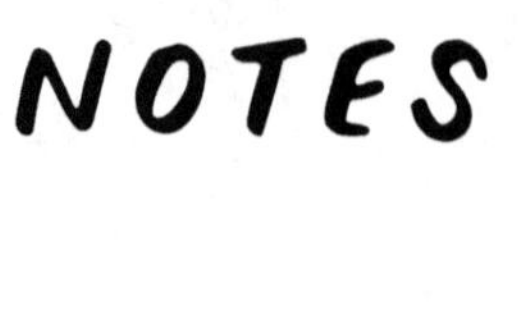

NOTES

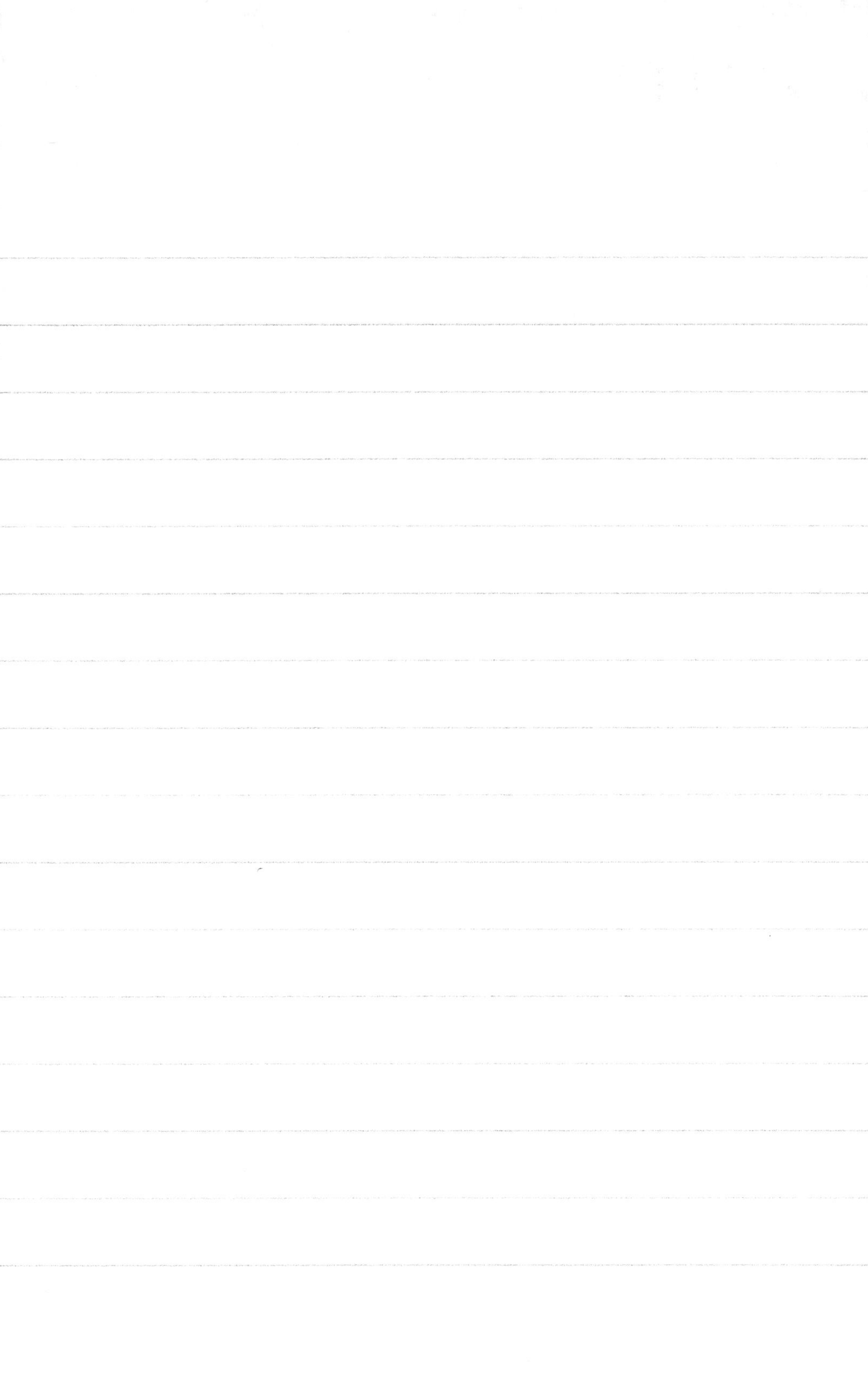

NOTES

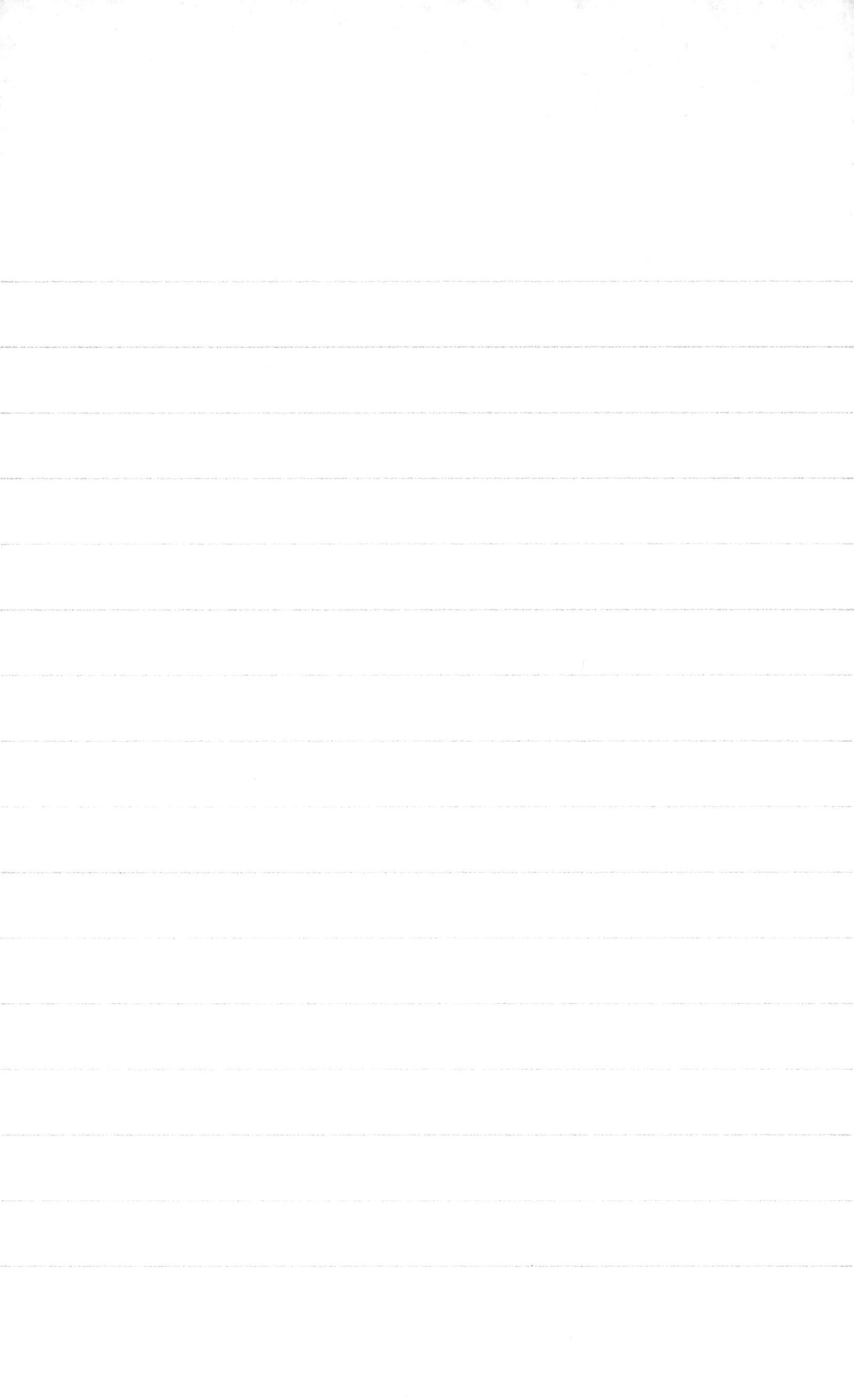